CONTENTS

INTRODUCTION

I don't believe that yoga should just be for the enlightened elite. Since engaging in an asana practice, I have personally experienced a number of benefits, physically and mentally. My mind is clearer; I've lost weight, and toned muscle.

After experiencing a number of different types of yoga classes, vinyasa, hot yoga, and hot power fusions, I put together a sequence that felt the best in my body. For me, the asana practice is about sweating, focusing, and clearing my mind. Practicing the same sequence each day has served as a moving meditation for me. I know what's coming next and all I have to think about as I am in each pose, is simply the pose itself, balance, muscle engagement, and form.

When I began teaching yoga, I looked for scripts, poses with cues, so that I could take some of the pressure off of being a new instructor. Leading a class through your first lesson can be stressful. I couldn't find anything on the Internet or marketplace to meet my needs. As I began writing this sequence and thinking about sharing it with other yoga practitioners and instructors, I realized that a script could become a useful tool. Not only does a script provide a sequence, but it also includes reminders of how to move in and out of each pose. *Flow Yoga Sequence: Advanced* is designed with ease of use and simplicity in mind. You have mastered *Flow Yoga Sequence*, now it is time to advance.

Flow Yoga Sequence: Advanced includes a Warm-Up Series, Sun Salutation, Warrior Series, Crescent Series, Chair Series, Balancing Series, Core Strengthening Series, Spine Strengthening Series, and a Cool-Down Series.

The Sanskrit names of each pose are included in the script. Get familiar with these, but don't use them until you are comfortable announcing them properly. I personally find an instructor who exclusively uses Sanskrit pose names to be a little ostentatious. Make sure that your class is accessible to your students.

You will notice that I repeat cues for each pose. I do so to establish a rhythm to be carried through the entire practice.

This is a moving practice that works for me. My students have enjoyed it, and I have personally been steadily losing weight since practicing this yoga sequence. I encourage you to customize *Flow Yoga Sequence: Advanced* to whatever feels best in your body, and use cues that are natural and authentic for you.

If you do decide to make changes to *Flow Yoga Sequence: Advanced*, I encourage you to do your research first. Make sure you are flowing breath to movement. Provide a good spinal warm-up and always twist right first in twisting poses. Maintain balance in your movements, and make sure that your sequence makes sense.

A fantastic way to make *Flow Yoga Sequence: Advanced* your own, without making actual changes to it, is by adding dialogue. Discuss breath and breath engagement in extended child's pose, and discuss the benefits of poses while you are in them. Guide your students out of final Savasana in a way that feels right for you. Educate yourself on the practice you teach, and share your knowledge and experience with your students.

For those of you who will not utilize the script, or no longer need to do so, the Flow Yoga Sequence: Advanced Cheat Sheet is a page you can find at the end of this book to tear out or refer to when you need quick reminders on the order of *Flow Yoga Sequence: Advanced.* Remember to offer modifications and practice safe alignment.

Practice in health and wellness.

FLOW YOGA SEQUENCE: ADVANCED

Warm-Up Series

Welcome to your advanced vinyasa yoga class.
Begin in Extended Child's Pose/ Balasana- Kneel on your
mat. Spread your knees wide. Bring your big toes to
touch. Place your forehead on the mat. Drop your hips
to your heels. Reach your arms overhead. Place your
palms on the mat. Engage your breath. Take a four
second inhale in through your nose. Take a four second
exhale out through your nose. Control your breath
throughout your practice.

(Inhale) Table-Top- Hold and breathe. Stack your
shoulders over your wrists. Stack your hips over your
knees. Keep a flat back.

(Inhale) Cow Pose/ Bitilasana- Drop your belly. Look up.
Lift your chest. Draw your shoulders away from your
ears.

(Exhale) Cat Pose/ Marjaryasana- Suck in your stomach.
Round your spine up. Relax the crown of your head
down towards the mat.

4

(Inhale) Cow Pose/ Bitilasana- Drop your belly. Lift your gaze. Lift your chest.

(Exhale) Cat Pose/ Marjaryasana- Suck in your stomach. Drop your head. Round your spine up.

(Inhale) Cow Pose/ Bitilasana- Drop your belly. Lift your gaze. Lift your chest.

(Exhale) Cat Pose/ Marjaryasana- Round your spine up. Drop your head. Suck in your stomach.

(Inhale) Table Top- Find a neutral spine. Hold and breathe.

Swimmers Pose- (Inhale) Extend your right arm straight ahead. Extend your left leg straight out from your hip. (Exhale) Round your spine. Connect your right elbow with your left knee. Suck in your stomach. (Inhale) Extend your right arm straight ahead. Extend your left leg straight out from your hip. (Exhale) Round your spine. Connect your right elbow with your left knee. Suck in your stomach.   (Inhale) Extend your right arm straight ahead. Extend your left leg straight out from your hip. (Exhale) Round your spine. Connect your right elbow with your left knee. Suck in your stomach. (Inhale) Extend your right arm straight ahead. Extend your left leg straight out from your hip.

(Exhale) Table Top- Release your hand and knee to the mat. Find a neutral spine.

Swimmers Pose- (Inhale) Extend your left arm straight ahead. Extend your right leg straight out from your hip. (Exhale) Round your spine. Connect your left elbow with your right knee. Suck in your stomach. (Inhale) Extend your left arm straight ahead. Extend your right leg straight out from your hip. (Exhale) Round your spine. Connect your left elbow with your right knee. Suck in your stomach. (Inhale) Extend your left arm straight ahead. Extend your right leg straight out from your hip. (Exhale) Round your spine. Connect your left elbow with your right knee. Suck in your stomach. (Inhale) Extend your left arm straight ahead. Extend your right leg straight out from your hip.

(Exhale) Table Top- Release your hand and knee to the mat. Find a neutral spine.

(Inhale) Prepare.

(Exhale) Downward Dog/ Adho Mukha Svanasana- Curl your toes under. Press down through your forefingers and your thumbs. Push your hips up high. Press your heels down towards the mat. Relax your neck. Point your tailbone up.

(Inhale) Walk your feet up to your hands.

(Exhale) Ragdoll Pose/ Uttanasana- Shift your weight to the balls of your feet. Fold forward at the hips. Grab opposite elbows. Relax your shoulders. Relax your head down towards the mat. Spread your toes. Keep your legs straight. Release your hands to the mat. Grab opposite elbows.

Release your hands to the mat. Toe-Heel your feet together.

Sun Salutation

(Inhale) Standing Savasana- Roll up one vertebra at a time to stand. (Exhale) Roll your shoulders up to your ears. Slide your shoulder blades together and down your back. Relax your arms to your sides. Face your palms forward.

(Inhale) Mountain Pose/ Tadasana- Ground down through your feet. Reach your arms up overhead. Relax your shoulders down. Roll your pinkies inward.

(Exhale) Mini Back-Bend- Lift your chest. Gaze up. Cactus your arms.

(Inhale) Mountain Pose/ Tadasana- Pull up on your knee caps. Reach up. Gaze forward.

(Exhale) Hands through Heart Center Forward Fold/ Uttanasana- Lead with your chest. Hinge at the hips. Fold with a flat back. Release your hands to the mat. Let your head hang heavy.

(Inhale) Halfway Lift/ Ardha Uttanasa- Lift your chest half way. Keep your back flat. Slide your shoulder blades together and down. Tuck your chin.

(Exhale) High to Low Plank/ Chaturanga Dandasana- Plant your hands. Step or float your feet back. Stack your shoulders over your wrists. Stay on the balls of your feet. Rock forward. Pin your elbows in. Lower halfway.

(Inhale) Upward Facing Dog/ Urdhva Mukha Svanasana- Flip the tops of your feet to the mat. Straighten your arms. Lift your chest. Lift your thighs off the mat.

(Exhale) Downward Dog/ Adho Mukha Svanasana- Curl your toes under. Press down through your forefingers and your thumbs. Push your hips up high. Press your heels down towards the mat. Relax your neck. Point your tailbone up.

(Inhale) Look up.

(Exhale) Step or float to the top of your mat. Bring your feet to touch.

(Inhale) Halfway Lift/ Ardha Uttanasa- Lift your chest half way. Keep your back flat. Slide your shoulder blades together and down. Tuck your chin.

(Exhale) Forward Fold/ Uttanasana- Hinge at the hips. Fold with a flat back. Release your hands to the mat. Let your head hang heavy.

Flow Sun Salutation

(Inhale) Mountain Pose/ Tadasana- Ground down through your feet. Reach your arms up overhead. Relax your shoulders down. Roll your pinkies inward.

(Exhale) Mini Back-Bend- Lift your chest. Gaze up. Cactus your arms.

(Inhale) Mountain Pose/ Tadasana- Pull up on your knee caps. Reach up. Gaze forward.

(Exhale) Hands through Heart Center Forward Fold/ Uttanasana- Lead with your chest. Hinge at the hips. Fold with a flat back. Release your hands to the mat. Let your head hang heavy.

(Inhale) Halfway Lift/ Ardha Uttanasa- Lift your chest half way. Keep your back flat. Slide your shoulder blades together and down. Tuck your chin.

(Exhale) High to Low Plank/ Chaturanga Dandasana-
Plant your hands. Step or float your feet back. Stack
your shoulders over your wrists. Stay on the balls of
your feet. Rock forward. Pin your elbows in. Lower
halfway.

(Inhale) Upward Facing Dog/ Urdhva Mukha Svanasana-
Flip the tops of your feet to the mat. Lift your chest.
Straighten your arms. Lift your thighs off the mat.

(Exhale) Downward Dog/ Adho Mukha Svanasana- Curl
your toes under. Press down through your forefingers
and your thumbs. Push your hips up high. Press your
heels down towards the mat. Relax your neck. Point
your tailbone up.

(Inhale) Look up.

(Exhale) Step or float to the top of your mat. Bring your
feet to touch.

(Inhale) Mountain Pose/ Tadasana- Ground down through your feet. Reach your arms up overhead. Relax your shoulders down. Roll your pinkies slightly inward.

(Exhale) Mini Back-Bend- Lift your chest. Gaze up. Cactus your arms.

(Inhale) Mountain Pose/ Tadasana- Pull up on your knee caps. Reach up. Gaze forward.

(Exhale) Hands through Heart Center Forward Fold/ Uttanasana- Lead with your chest. Hinge at the hips. Fold with a flat back. Release your hands to the floor. Let your head hang heavy.

(Inhale) Halfway Lift/ Ardha Uttanasa- Lift your chest half way. Keep your back flat. Slide your shoulder blades together and down. Tuck your chin.

(Exhale) High to Low Plank/ Chaturanga Dandasana-
Plant your hands. Step or float your feet back. Stack
your shoulders over your wrists. Stay on the balls of
your feet. Rock forward. Pin your elbows in. Lower
halfway.

(Inhale) Upward Facing Dog/ Urdhva Mukha Svanasana-
Flip the tops of your feet to the mat. Straighten your
arms. Lift your chest. Lift your thighs off the mat.

(Exhale) Downward Dog/ Adho Mukha Svanasana- Curl
your toes under. Press down through your forefingers
and your thumbs. Push your hips up high. Press your
heels down towards the mat. Relax your neck and look
through your legs. Point your tailbone up.

Warrior Series

(Inhale) Right leg high.

(Exhale) Low Lunge- Step between your hands.

(Inhale) Warrior II/ Virabhadrasana II- Point your front toes forward. Spin your back foot parallel with the back of your mat. Open your hips to the side. Lift your arms to shoulder height. Put a 90 degree bend in your front knee. Gaze over your front hand.

(Exhale) Humble Warrior- Interlace your fingers behind your back. Expand your chest. Hinge forward at your hips. Lead with your chest. Point your interlaced fingers straight up. Bring your right shoulder to the inside of your front knee.

(Inhale) Warrior II/ Virabhadrasana II- Rise up. Release your grip. Lift your arms to shoulder height. Keep a 90 degree bend in your front knee. Gaze over your front hand.

(Exhale) Extended Side Angle/ Utthita Parsvakonasana-
Reach your front arm forward and down. Reach your
back arm up. Gaze up.

(Inhale) Reverse Warrior/ Parivrtta Virabhadrasana II-
Reach your back arm down. Reach your front arm up.
Gaze up. Keep your front knee bent. Keep your back
leg straight.

(Exhale) Triangle Pose/ Trikonasana- Straighten your
front leg. Keep your back leg straight. Reach your front
arm forward and down. Reach your back arm up. Open
your chest.

(Inhale) Reverse Triangle- Reach your back arm down.
Reach your front arm up. Gaze up. Keep both legs
straight.

(Exhale) High to Low Plank/ Chaturanga Dandasana-
Cartwheel your arms down. Plant your hands. Step or
float your feet back. Stack your shoulders over your
wrists. Stay on the balls of your feet. Rock forward. Pin
your elbows in. Lower halfway.

(Inhale) Upward Facing Dog/ Urdhva Mukha Svanasana-
Flip the tops of your feet to the mat. Straighten your
arms. Lift your chest. Lift your thighs off the mat.

(Exhale) Downward Dog/ Adho Mukha Svanasana- Curl
your toes under. Press down through your forefingers
and your thumbs. Push your hips up high. Press your
heels down towards the mat. Relax your neck. Point
your tailbone up.

(Inhale) Left leg high.

(Exhale) Low Lunge- Step between your hands.

(Inhale) Warrior II/ Virabhadrasana II- Point your front
toes forward. Spin your back foot parallel with the back
of your mat. Open your hips to the side. Lift your arms
to shoulder height. Put a 90 degree bend in your front
knee. Gaze over your front hand.

(Exhale) Humble Warrior- Interlace your fingers behind your back. Expand your chest. Hinge forward at your hips. Lead with your chest. Point your interlaced fingers straight up. Bring your right shoulder to the inside of your front knee.

(Inhale) Warrior II/ Virabhadrasana II- Rise up. Release your grip. Lift your arms to shoulder height. Keep a 90 degree bend in your front knee. Gaze over your front hand.

(Exhale) Extended Side Angle/ Utthita Parsvakonasana- Reach your front arm forward and down. Reach your back arm up. Gaze up.

(Inhale) Reverse Warrior/ Parivrtta Virabhadrasana II- Reach your back arm down. Reach your front arm up. Gaze up. Keep your front knee bent. Keep your back leg straight.

(Exhale) Triangle Pose/ Trikonasana- Straighten your front leg. Keep your back leg straight. Reach your front arm forward and down. Reach your back arm up. Open your chest.

(Inhale) Reverse Triangle- Reach your back arm down. Reach your front arm up. Gaze up. Keep both legs straight.

(Exhale) High to Low Plank/ Chaturanga Dandasana- Cartwheel your arms down. Plant your hands. Step or float your feet back. Stack your shoulders over your wrists. Stay on the balls of your feet. Rock forward. Pin your elbows in. Lower halfway.

(Inhale) Upward Facing Dog/ Urdhva Mukha Svanasana- Flip the tops of your feet to the mat. Straighten your arms. Lift your chest. Lift your thighs off the mat.

(Exhale) Downward Dog/ Adho Mukha Svanasana- Curl your toes under. Press down through your forefingers and your thumbs. Push your hips up high. Press your heels down towards the mat. Relax your neck. Point your tailbone up.

Flow Warrior Series (Add Standing Straddle Bend, Remove Humble Warrior)

(Inhale) Right leg high.

(Exhale) Low Lunge- Step between your hands.

(Inhale) Warrior II/ Virabhadrasana II- Point your front toes forward. Spin your back foot parallel with the back of your mat. Open your hips to the side. Lift your arms to shoulder height. Put a 90 degree bend in your front knee. Gaze over your front hand.

(Exhale) Extended Side Angle/ Utthita Parsvakonasana- Reach your front arm forward and down. Reach your back arm up. Gaze up.

(Inhale) Reverse Warrior/ Parivrtta Virabhadrasana II- Reach your back arm down. Reach your front arm up. Gaze up. Keep your front knee bent. Keep your back leg straight.

(Exhale) Triangle Pose/ Trikonasana- Straighten your front leg. Keep your back leg straight. Reach your front arm forward and down. Reach your back arm up. Open your chest.

(Inhale) Reverse Triangle- Reach your back arm down. Reach your front arm up. Gaze up. Keep both legs straight.

(Exhale) Warrior II/ Virabhadrasana II- Point your front toes forward. Spin your back foot parallel with the back of your mat. Open your hips to the side. Lift your arms to shoulder height. Put a 90 degree bend in your front knee. Gaze over your front hand.

(Inhale) Straighten both legs. Pivot your right foot so it's parallel to the left. Lift your chest. Look forward.

(Exhale) Standing Straddle Bend/ Prasarita Padottanasana- Hinge at the hips. Lower with a flat back. Grab the outside of your feet or ankles or release your hands to the mat.

(Inhale) Rise up. Extend your arms straight out from your shoulders to your sides. Use your core and inner thigh strength to rise.

(Exhale) Warrior II/ Virabhadrasana II- Pivot your right toes to the top of your mat. Keep your back foot parallel with the back of your mat. Open your hips to the side. Keep your arms at shoulder height. Put a 90 degree bend in your front knee. Gaze over your front hand.

(Inhale) Prepare.

(Exhale) High to Low Plank/ Chaturanga Dandasana- Cartwheel your arms down. Plant your hands. Step or float your feet back. Stack your shoulders over your wrists. Stay on the balls of your feet. Rock forward. Pin your elbows in. Lower halfway.

(Inhale) Upward Facing Dog/ Urdhva Mukha Svanasana- Flip the tops of your feet to the mat. Straighten your arms. Lift your chest. Lift your thighs off the mat.

(Exhale) Downward Dog/ Adho Mukha Svanasana- Curl your toes under. Press down through your forefinger and your thumb. Push your hips up high. Press your heels down towards the mat. Relax your neck. Point your tailbone up.

(Inhale) Left leg high.

(Exhale) Low Lunge- Step between your hands.

(Inhale) Warrior II/ Virabhadrasana II- Point your front toes forward. Spin your back foot parallel with the back of your mat. Open your hips to the side. Lift your arms to shoulder height. Put a 90 degree bend in your front knee. Gaze over your front hand.

(Exhale) Extended Side Angle/ Utthita Parsvakonasana- Reach your front arm forward and down. Reach your back arm up. Gaze up.

(Inhale) Reverse Warrior/ Parivrtta Virabhadrasana II-
Reach your back arm down. Reach your front arm up.
Gaze up. Keep your front knee bent. Keep your back leg
straight.

(Exhale) Triangle Pose/ Trikonasana- Straighten your
front leg. Keep your back leg straight. Reach your front
arm forward and down. Reach your back arm up. Open
your chest.

(Inhale) Reverse Triangle- Reach your back arm down.
Reach your front arm up. Gaze up. Keep both legs
straight.

(Exhale) Warrior II/ Virabhadrasana II- Point your front
toes forward. Spin your back foot parallel with the back
of your mat. Open your hips to the side. Lift your arms
to shoulder height. Put a 90 degree bend in your front
knee. Gaze over your front hand.

(Inhale) Straighten both legs. Pivot your left foot so it's
parallel to the right. Lift your chest. Look forward.

(Exhale) Standing Straddle Bend/ Prasarita
Padottanasana- Interlace your fingers behind your back
for a chest expansion. Keep a micro bend in your
elbows. Hinge at the hips. Lower with a flat back.

(Inhale) Rise up. Use your core and inner thigh strength
to rise.

(Exhale) Warrior II/ Virabhadrasana II- Release your
grip. Point your front toes forward. Keep your back foot
parallel with the back of your mat. Open your hips to
the side. Lift your arms to shoulder height. Put a 90
degree bend in your front knee. Gaze over your front
hand.

(Inhale) Prepare.

(Exhale) High to Low Plank/ Chaturanga Dandasana-
Cartwheel your arms down. Plant your hands. Step or
float your feet back. Stack your shoulders over your
wrists. Stay on the balls of your feet. Rock forward. Pin
your elbows in. Lower halfway.

(Inhale) Upward Facing Dog/ Urdhva Mukha Svanasana-
Flip the tops of your feet to the mat. Straighten your
arms. Lift your chest. Lift your thighs off the mat.

(Exhale) Downward Dog/ Adho Mukha Svanasana- Curl
your toes under. Press down through your forefinger
and your thumb. Push your hips up high. Press your
heels down towards the mat. Relax your neck. Point
your tailbone up.

Crescent Series

(Inhale) Right leg high.

(Exhale) Low Lunge- Step between your hands.

(Inhale) Crescent Lunge/ Anjaneyasana- Hold and breathe. Keep your feet hip distance apart. Put a 90 degree bend in your front knee. Keep your back leg straight. Stay on the ball of your back foot. Lift your chest. Reach your arms overhead. Relax your shoulders.

(Exhale) Revolved Crescent Lunge/ Parivrtta Anjaneyasna- Bring your hands to heart center. Twist your torso to the right. Place your left elbow on the outside of your right knee. Draw your shoulder blades together.

(Inhale) Prepare.

(Exhale) Runner's Lunge- Release your hands to the mat. Walk your front toes to the top outside corner of your mat. Stack your knee above your ankle. Drop your back knee to the mat. Lower to your forearms.

(Inhale) Prepare.

(Exhale) High Plank- Straighten your arms. Stack your shoulders over your wrists. Step your right foot back to meet your left.

(Inhale) Side Plank- Hold and breathe. Bring your feet together. Roll to the outer edge of your left foot. Raise your right arm high. Drop to your left knee to the mat if needed. Lift your hips. Lift your chest.

(Exhale) High to Low Plank/ Chaturanga Dandasana- Plant your right hand and foot on the mat. Stack your shoulders over your wrists. Stay on the balls of your feet. Rock forward. Pin your elbows in. Lower halfway.

(Inhale) Upward Facing Dog/ Urdhva Mukha Svanasana- Flip the tops of your feet to the mat. Straighten your arms. Lift your chest. Lift your thighs off the mat.

(Exhale) Downward Dog/ Adho Mukha Svanasana- Curl your toes under. Press down through your forefinger and your thumb. Push your hips up high. Press your heels down towards the mat. Relax your neck. Point your tailbone up.

(Inhale) Left leg high.

(Exhale) Low Lunge- Step between your hands.

(Inhale) Crescent Lunge/ Anjaneyasana- Hold and breathe. Keep your feet hip distance apart. Put a 90 degree bend in your front knee. Keep your back leg straight. Stay on the ball of your back foot. Lift your chest. Reach your arms overhead. Relax your shoulders.

(Exhale) Revolved Crescent Lunge/ Parivrtta
Anjaneyasna- Bring your hands to heart center. Twist
your torso to the left. Place your right elbow on the
outside of your left knee. Draw your shoulder blades
together.

(Inhale) Prepare.

(Exhale) Runner's Lunge- Release your hands to the
mat. Walk your front toes to the top outside corner of
your mat. Stack your knee above your ankle. Drop your
back knee to the mat. Lower to your forearms.

(Inhale) Prepare.

(Exhale) High Plank- Straighten your arms. Stack your
shoulders over your wrists. Step your right foot back to
meet your left.

(Inhale) Side Plank- Hold and breathe. Bring your feet
together. Roll to the outer edge of your right foot.
Raise your right arm high. Drop to your right knee to
the mat if needed. Lift your hips. Lift your chest.

(Exhale) High to Low Plank/ Chaturanga Dandasana-
Plant your left hand and foot on the mat. Stack your
shoulders over your wrists. Stay on the balls of your
feet. Rock forward. Pin your elbows in. Lower halfway.

(Inhale) Upward Facing Dog/ Urdhva Mukha Svanasana-
Flip the tops of your feet to the mat. Straighten your
arms. Lift your chest. Lift your thighs off the mat.

(Exhale) Downward Dog/ Adho Mukha Svanasana- Curl
your toes under. Press down through your forefinger
and your thumb. Push your hips up high. Press your
heels down towards the mat. Relax your neck. Point
your tailbone up.

Chair Series

(Inhale) Look up.

(Exhale) Step or float to the top of your mat.

(Inhale) Chair Pose/ Utkatasana- Step your feet together. Shift your weight to your heels. Sit your hips down deep. Reach your arms up overhead. Turn your pinkies in. Relax your shoulders away from your ears.

(Exhale) Prayer Twist- Parivrtta Utkatasana- Bring your hands to heart center. Twist your torso to the right. Bring your left elbow to the outside of your right knee. Open your chest to the side. Spread your arms. Reach your right arm up. Reach your left arm down.

(Inhale) Chair Pose/ Utkatasana- Shift your weight to your heels. Sit your hips down deep. Reach your arms up overhead. Turn your pinkies in. Relax your shoulders away from your ears.

(Exhale) Hands through Heart Center Forward Fold/Uttanasana- Lead with your chest. Hinge at the hips. Fold with a flat back. Release your hands to the mat. Let your head hang heavy.

(Inhale) Halfway Lift/ Ardha Uttanasa- Lift your chest half way. Keep your back flat. Slide your shoulder blades together and down. Tuck your chin.

(Exhale) Gorilla Pose- Padahastasana- Separate your feet hip width distance apart. Hinge forward from your hips. Place your hands under your feet so your toes brush your wrists. Relax your head down. Bow your elbows out.

Release your hands. Toe-Heel your feet together.

(Inhale) Chair Pose/ Utkatasana- Shift your weight to your heels. Sit your hips down deep. Reach your arms up overhead. Turn your pinkies in. Relax your shoulders away from your ears.

(Exhale) Prayer Twist- Parivrtta Utkatasana- Bring your hands to heart center. Twist your torso to the left. Bring your right elbow to the outside of your left knee. Open your chest to the side. Spread your arms. Reach your left arm up. Reach your right arm down.

(Inhale) Chair Pose/ Utkatasana- Shift your weight to your heels. Sit your hips down deep. Reach your arms up overhead. Turn your pinkies in. Relax your shoulders away from your ears.

(Exhale) Hands through Heart Center Forward Fold/ Uttanasana- Lead with your chest. Hinge at the hips. Fold with a flat back. Release your hands to the mat. Let your head hang heavy.

(Inhale) Halfway Lift/ Ardha Uttanasa- Lift your chest half way. Keep your back flat. Slide your shoulder blades together and down. Tuck your chin.

(Exhale) Hands to Feet Pose- Padahastasana- Separate your feet hip width distance apart. Hinge forward from your hips. Grab your big toes with your pointer finger and your middle finger. Relax your head down. Bow your elbows out.

Release your hands. Toe-Heel your feet together.

(Inhale) Chair Pose/ Utkatasana- Shift your weight to your heels. Sit your hips down deep. Reach your arms up overhead. Turn your pinkies in. Relax your shoulders away from your ears.

Balancing Series

(Exhale) Eagle Pose to Eagle Arm Airplane/ Garudasana-
Touch your palms overhead. Swing your right arm
under and around your left arm. Cross at your elbows
and your wrists. Wrap your right leg up and over your
left leg. Double wrap at the calf. Line up your knees
and your elbows. Tuck your pelvis. Straighten your
back. Find your gaze over your hands. (Inhale) Shift
your weight to your standing leg. (Exhale) Unwrap your
right leg. Hinge forward at your hips. Extend your right
leg straight back. Move your elbows away from your
chest.

(Inhale) Chair Pose/ Utkatasana- Unwrap your arms.
Step your feet together. Shift your weight to your
heels. Sit your hips down deep. Reach your arms up
overhead. Turn your pinkies in. Relax your shoulders
away from your ears.

(Exhale) Eagle Pose to Eagle Arm Airplane/ Garudasana-
Touch your palms overhead. Swing your left arm under
and around your right arm. Cross at your elbows and
your wrists. Wrap your left leg up and over your right
leg. Double wrap at the calf. Line up your knees and
your elbows. Tuck your pelvis. Straighten your back.
Find your gaze over your hands. (Inhale) Shift your
weight to your standing leg. (Exhale) Unwrap your left
leg. Hinge forward at your hips. Extend your left leg
straight back. Move your elbows away from your chest.

(Inhale) Mountain Pose/ Tadasana- Unwrap your arms.
Step your feet together. Ground down through your
feet. Reach your arms up overhead. Relax your
shoulders. Roll your pinkies slightly inward.

(Exhale) Dancer's Pose/ Natarajasana- Bring your right
elbow to your right side body. Bend your right knee.
Grab your foot from the inside. Squeeze your knees
together. Kick up with your right foot. Reach up with
your left hand. Lift your chest. Keep your hips square
to the front of the room.

(Inhale) Mountain Pose/ Tadasana- Release your foot. Ground down through your feet. Reach your arms up overhead. Relax your shoulders. Roll your pinkies slightly inward.

(Exhale) Dancer's Pose/ Natarajasana- Bring your left elbow to your left side body. Bend your left knee. Grab your foot from the inside. Squeeze your knees together. Kick up with your left foot. Reach up with your right hand. Lift your chest. Keep your hips square to the front of the room.

(Inhale) Mountain Pose/ Tadasana- Release your foot. Ground down through your feet. Reach your arms up overhead. Relax your shoulders. Roll your pinkies slightly inward.

(Exhale) Tree Pose/ Vrksasana- Hands to heart center. Place your right foot on your ankle, calf, or inner thigh. Lift your chest. Relax your shoulders. Option to lift your arms and grow your branches.

(Inhale) Mountain Pose/ Tadasana- Drop your right foot
to meet your left. Ground down through your feet.
Reach your arms up overhead. Relax your shoulders.
Roll your pinkies slightly inward.

(Exhale) Tree Pose/ Vrksasana- Hands to heart center.
Place your left foot on your ankle, calf, or inner thigh.
Lift your chest. Relax your shoulders. Option to lift
your arms and grow your branches.

(Inhale) Mountain Pose/ Tadasana- Drop your left foot
to meet your right. Ground down through your feet.
Reach your arms up overhead. Relax your shoulders.
Roll your pinkies slightly inward.

(Exhale) Hands through Heart Center Forward Fold/
Uttanasana- Lead with your chest. Hinge at the hips.
Fold with a flat back. Release your hands to the mat.
Let your head hang heavy.

(Inhale) Halfway Lift/ Ardha Uttanasa- Lift your chest
half way. Keep your back flat. Slide your shoulder
blades together and down. Tuck your chin.

(Exhale) Crow Pose/ Bakasana- Plant your hands on the floor shoulder width apart. Spread your fingers wide. Tilt your body forwards and bend your elbows. Place your knees on your triceps. Lift one foot off the ground, then the other.

(Exhale) High to Low Plank/ Chaturanga Dandasana- Plant your hands. Step or float your feet back. Stack your shoulders over your wrists. Stay on the balls of your feet. Rock forward. Pin your elbows in. Lower halfway.

(Inhale) Upward Facing Dog/ Urdhva Mukha Svanasana- Flip the tops of your feet to the mat. Straighten your arms. Lift your chest. Lift your thighs off the mat.

(Exhale) Downward Dog/ Adho Mukha Svanasana- Curl your toes under. Press down through your forefinger and your thumb. Push your hips up high. Press your heels down towards the mat. Relax your neck. Point your tailbone up.

(Inhale) Right leg high.

(Exhale) Half Pigeon/ Eka Pada Rajakapotasana- Bring your right knee to your right wrist. Bring your foot towards your left wrist. Drop down to your back knee. Flatten your back leg down. Walk your hands up to the top of your mat and come down to your forearms.

(Inhale) Proud Pigeon- Walk your hands back towards your hips. Puff up your chest.

(Exhale) Quad Stretch- Bend your left knee. Grab your left foot with your right hand.

(Inhale) Proud Pigeon- Release your foot. Plant your hand.

(Exhale) Downward Dog/ Adho Mukha Svanasana- Step your right foot back to meet your left foot. Curl your toes under. Press down through your forefinger and your thumb. Push your hips up high. Press your heels down towards the mat. Relax your neck. Point your tailbone up.

(Inhale) Left leg high.

(Exhale) Half Pigeon/ Eka Pada Rajakapotasana- Bring your left knee to your left wrist. Bring your foot towards your right wrist. Drop down to your back knee. Flatten your back leg down. Walk your hands up to the top of your mat and come down to your forearms.

(Inhale) Proud Pigeon- Walk your hands back to your hips. Puff up your chest.

(Exhale) Quad Stretch- Bend your right knee. Grab your right foot with your left hand.

(Inhale) Proud Pigeon- Release your foot. Plant your hand.

(Exhale) Downward Dog/ Adho Mukha Svanasana-   Step your left foot back to meet your right foot. Curl your toes under. Press down through your forefinger and your thumb. Push your hips up high. Press your heels down towards the mat. Relax your neck. Point your tailbone up.

(Inhale) Step or float to the top of your mat.

(Exhale) Cross your ankles and have a seat.

Core Strengthening Series

Boat Pose/ Navasana- Bend your knees. Place your feet flat on the floor. Lean back slightly. Place your hands behind your thighs. Lift your feet off the floor. Float your hands to your sides. Straighten your legs.

Full Body Stretch- Lie flat on your back. Stretch your arms up. Stretch your legs out.

Sarahbi Ab Ladder- Lie on your back. Lift your legs straight up. Keep your entire back on the mat. Lift your legs straight up. Lower your legs toe inches and hold. Lower your legs another two inches and hold. Lower your legs two inches above the mat and hold. Lift your leg two inches and hold. Lift your legs another two inches and hold. Lift your legs straight up. Stack your right foot over your left foot. Keep your legs straight. Lower your legs two inches and hold. Lower your legs another two inches and hold. Lower your legs two inches above the mat and hold. Lift your legs two inches and hold. Lift your legs another two inches and hold. Lift your legs straight up and switch your feet. Stack your left foot over your right foot. Lower your legs two inches and hold. Lower your legs another two inches and hold. Lower your legs two inches above the mat and hold. Lift your legs two inches and hold. Lift your legs another two inches and hold. Lift your legs straight up the wall. Slowly lower your legs all the way down.

Full Body Stretch- Stretch your arms up. Stretch your legs out.

Legs up the Wall Cherry Pickers/ Viparita Karani- Lie on your back. Lift your legs straight up. Keep your entire back on the mat. Lift your shoulders off the mat. Keep your legs straight. Reach for your left foot with your right hand, then your right foot with your left hand. Alternate back and forth, exhaling as your lift.

Full Body Stretch- Lie on your back. Stretch your arms up. Stretch your legs out.

SAM SARAHBI

Spine Strengthening Series

Come to the front of your mat. Lie on your stomach.

Cobra Pose/ Bhujangasana- Bring your chin to center.
Zip your legs together. Bring the heels of your hands
towards your top ribs. Look forward. (Inhale) With very
little weight in your hands, lift your chest. (Exhale)
Press your feet into the mat. (Inhale) Place a little more
weight into your hands and peel another rib off the
mat.

(Exhale) Release to the mat. Lay your left ear on the
mat. Release your arms to your side. Let your heels fall
apart.

Bow Pose/ Dhanurasana- Bring your chin back to center.
Bend your knees. Grab your feet from the outsides.
Squeeze your knees back together. (Inhale) Lift your
chest. (Exhale) Kick into your hands. (Inhale) Kick a
little higher.

(Exhale) Release to the mat. Lay your right ear on the mat. Release your arms to your sides. Let your heels fall apart.

Push up to table top position. Stand on your knees at the center of your mat. Separate your knees hip width distance apart.

Camel Pose/ Ustrasana- Place your hands on your lower back. Point your fingers down. Squeeze your elbows together. (Inhale) Lift your gaze. Lift your chest. (Exhale) Push your hips forward. Walk your gaze back. Grab one heel, then the other. Keep pushing your hips forward. If you've reclined, place one hand, then the other on your lower back as you come back up. Take a seat on your heels.

Spin your legs out in front of you. Sit on your sitz bones. Hover your arms out to your sides. Slowly recline with control to lie flat on your back.

Wheel Pose/ Urdhva Dhanuasana- Bring your heels near your seat. Plant your feet hip width distance apart. Bend your elbows. Plant your hands behind at the sides of your head. (Inhale) Raise your hips. (Exhale) Push your arms straight.

Lower down to the mat. Stretch your legs out.

Cool Down Series

Double Exhale Sit-Up- Zip your legs together. Reach your arms overhead. Cross your thumbs. (Inhale) Prepare. (Exhale) Sit up. (Exhale) Fold over.

Seated Forward Fold/ Paschimottanasana- Grab your big toes with your middle and your pointer fingers. Bend your knees as much as necessary to make a chest to thigh connection. Keep a flat back. Slowly push your heels out. Keep your chest to thigh connection.

Release your toes. Straighten your legs out in front of you. Hover your arms out to your side. Recline with control. Lie flat on your back.

Shoulder Stand/ Salamba Sarvangasana- Lift your legs to legs up the wall pose. Option to stay here. Option to lift your hips off the floor. Support your lower back with your hands. Plant your elbows on the mat. Reach your legs straight up. Push your toes away from your face. Push your hips towards your face. Keep pressure off of your neck.

Ear Pinning Pose/ Karnapidasana – Bend your knees. Bring them to the outside of your ears. Keep the weight in your shoulders and off of your neck.

Plow Pose/ Halasana- Straighten your legs. Reach them back to touch the floor behind you. Plant your palms on the mat straight ahead.

Happy Baby Pose/ Ananda Balasana- Roll down onto your back with control. Grab the insides of your feet. Pull your knees towards your armpits. Rock gently from side to side, massaging your spine.

Supine Twist/ Jathara Parivartanasan- Relax your left leg to the mat. Squeeze your right knee into your right armpit. With your left hand, gently guide your knee across your body. Extend your right arm out. Gaze right.

Come back to center.

Supine Twist/ Jathara Parivartanasan- Relax your right leg to the mat. Squeeze your left knee into your left armpit. With your right hand, gently guide your knee across your body. Extend your left arm out. Gaze left.

Hug both of your knees into your chest. Keep your entire back flat on the mat. (Inhale) Bring your head to your knees. Squeeze tightly into a ball.

(Exhale) Corpse Pose/ Savasana- Relax your legs out in front of you. Let your toes fall apart. Relax your arms at your sides. Close your eyes.

FLOW YOGA SEQUENCE: ADVANCED CHEAT SHEET

WARM-UP
EXTENDED CHILD
COW/CAT (X3)
SWIMMERS
DOWN DOG
RAGDOLL

SUN SALUTATION (X3)

WARRIOR (X2 (R/L))
WARRIOR II
HUMBLE
WARRIOR II
EXTENDED SIDE
REVERSE WARRIOR
TRIANGLE
REVERSE TRIANGLE
(ADD STRADDLE,
REMOVE HUMBLE @
FLOWS)

CRESCENT (1X (R/L)
CRESCENT LUNGE
REVOLVE CRESC LNG
RUNNER'S LUNGE
SIDE PLANK

CHAIR
CHAIR
PRAYER TWIST (R)
GORILLA
CHAIR
PRAYER TWIST (L)
HANDS TO FEET

BALANCING
EAGLE (R/L)
DANCER (R/L)
TREE (R/L)
CROW
PIGEON (R/L)

CORE
BOAT
SARAHBI AB LADDER
LEGS UP WALL PICKER

SPINE
COBRA
BOW
CAMEL
WHEEL

COOL-DOWN
SEATED FWD FOLD
SHOULDER STAND
PLOW
HAPPY BABY
SUPINE TWIST (R/L)
CORPSE

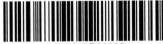

21623617R00036

Printed in Great Britain
by Amazon